What Christians Should Know About...

Sickness and Healing

Ed Harding

Sovereign World

Copyright © 1997 Ed Harding

All rights reserved. No part of this publication may be reproduced, stored in a retrieval system, or transmitted in any form or by any means, electronic, mechanical, photocopying, recording or otherwise, without the prior written consent of the publisher.

Short extracts may be quoted for review purposes.

ISBN: 1 85240 211 3

Scripture quotations are taken from the HOLY BIBLE, NEW INTERNATIONAL VERSION. Copyright © 1973, 1978, 1984 by International Bible Society. Used by permission.

SOVEREIGN WORLD LIMITED
P.O. Box 777, Tonbridge, Kent TN11 9XT, England.

Typeset and printed in the UK by Sussex Litho Ltd, Chichester, West Sussex.

About the Author

Ed Harding believes passionately in divine healing and the full restoration of all the gifts and ministries God wants in the Body of Christ. He has been taking ministry teams overseas for a number of years especially to India, to preach the gospel with signs following.

Ed has seen a number of spectacular miracles with many people healed and delivered from demonic oppression, and he has also seen many people that have not been healed. He wants to extend the teaching ministry through books such as this to see God's people come into full understanding and blessing.

Ed is also the author of QUENCH NOT THE SPIRIT, written some years ago at a time of resistance to the move of God.

He lives in West Sussex with his wife and three children, and has moved out of local Church leadership to be free to travel and teach more widely.

Contents

	Introduction	7
1	Genesis and the Fall	9
2	The Three Sources of Sickness	13
	a) The Fall – physical	
	b) Satan – spiritual	
	c) God – judgement	
3	The Effects of the Curse	19
	a) On a nation	
	b) On a family	
	c) On an individual	
4	Christ our Redeemer	21
5	Physical or Spiritual?	25
6	Biblical Methods of Healing	29
	a) The Laying on of hands	
	b) Summoning the Elders	
	c) Gifts of healing/special meetings	
7	Blockages to Healing	31
8	What to do if You're Sick	33
	Finally... never give up	37

Introduction

Healing is probably the most controversial and contentious issue which Christians face in the Church today. You may well know someone who says they have been healed by God's supernatural power. You will also, most likely, know of those with good Christian character who have not recovered despite much prayer and intercession on their behalf. At one extreme there are those who believe and teach that everyone should be healed if only they learned how to appropriate the scriptures and had enough faith. At the other extreme there are those who believe that God does not intervene to heal supernaturally today, and to teach that He does raises false hopes. Indeed, worse than that, they say it is a cruel deception which leaves the victim in unreality and quite unprepared for death.

The shock then affects the family. What if they had prayed more? Did they have too little faith? Why did God ignore their prayers? What about all those promises in the Bible? If you then consider all the apparent unjust suffering of, for example, children with terminal illnesses, where is God in it all? Where is His love and compassion?

In this short book we will try to address some of these issues to see precisely what Scripture teaches, both for the believer and the unbeliever.

As a personal introduction I have, over some 28 years as a Christian, been healed by God of conditions for which I was receiving specialist medical treatment, seen God do some spectacular miracles, and also witnessed the death of good solid Christian friends.

Should everybody expect to be healed in all circumstances or is healing conditional? If so what are the conditions? Or did it all cease with the apostles?

But before we address such questions we have to go right back to the beginning. We need to know where sickness comes from. As is so often the case, the key lies in Genesis.

1

Genesis and the Fall

Just as you will never understand your salvation properly until you understand the Fall of Man, equally I believe you need to see what precisely happened at that time when the whole human race fell under God's judgement, to understand sickness, the effects of sin and how God made provision for Adam and mankind.

In Genesis 2:17 Adam is forbidden to eat of the tree of the knowledge of good and evil *"for when you eat of it you will surely die"* (NIV). Literally it translates 'dying you shall die'. Up to that point Adam had eternal life, a perfect disease-free body created for eternity, and had he not sinned would still be here now! Incidentally that's why God will create a new heaven **and** a new earth, because it's the perfect environment for man and is part of the divine plan of restoration of all things. Those who think only heaven is our final destination are in for a most wonderful surprise!

The effects of the Fall of Man were devastating:

> To the serpent God said *"**Cursed** are you above all the livestock."* (Genesis 3:14)

> To the woman God said *"I will greatly increase your **pains** in childbearing; with **pain** you will give birth to children."* (Genesis 3:16)

> To Adam God said *"**Cursed** is the ground because of you; through **painful** toil you will eat of it... By the sweat of your brow you will eat your food until you return to the ground."* (Genesis 3:17,19)

Hence the whole human race came under God's judgement, with toil, sweat, tears and finally death. Man had fallen. Worse was to come.

Initially, if you read Genesis 5, you'll see that Adam lived to be 930 years old (verse 5), Seth lived to 912 years (verse 8), Enoch 905 (verse 11), Kenan 910 (verse 14), and so it goes on, naming ages of 895, 962, 365 (Enoch who never died), 969 and 777 years. Then there is a further phase of judgement – God shortens life to 120 years, basically because of sin. Note what God says:

> *"My Spirit will not contend with man for ever, for he is mortal; his days will be a hundred and twenty years."*
> (Genesis 6:3)

Why? Verse 11 tells us *"Now the earth was corrupt in God's sight and was full of violence.."* As a consequence, all of mankind was destroyed in a global flood over the whole earth, together with all the animals apart from those in the ark. That judgement had a dramatic effect on the world's climate, eradicating huge areas of vegetation, and causing many species of animals to die out.

Although we're perhaps more familiar with God's promise never to flood the earth again God made another promise:

> *"Never again will I curse the ground because of man, even though every inclination of his heart is evil from childhood."*
> (Genesis 8:21)

This expresses His heart. God must judge sin, but He wants to bless.

You may wonder what this has to do with healing, but unless you diagnose the root cause of sickness correctly you won't apply the correct remedy. Sickness was part of the judgement at the Fall. By the time of King David God had shortened life even more:

> *"The length of our days is seventy years – or eighty if we have the strength."* (Psalm 90:10)

In the nineteen-nineties the average age span has in fact now risen to over eighty, largely due to medical technology prolonging life, rather than natural strength as in David's day. Long life is seen as a blessing in the Bible, a short life a curse. That's not just a promise linked to the commandment to honour your father and mother, but the theme runs right through Scripture. Perhaps the clearest expression of God's intention is in Isaiah 65:20 which describes the reign of Christ on earth:

> *"Never again will there be in it an infant that lives but a few days, or an old man who does not live out his years; he who dies at a hundred will be thought a mere youth;* ***he who fails to reach a hundred will be considered accursed.****"*

So where is this all leading? It shows that **all** of mankind is still under the curse of a shortened life, the ageing process, decay and finally death. You may wonder why I say that everyone is under the curse of decay, but the answer is actually very simple. You cannot die without a bodily malfunction. It is simply impossible! Whether you are shot in a war or die in your sleep the doctor writing your death certificate has to state a cause of death. Parts of the body stop functioning – that's how you die! The wonderful truth about our new resurrection bodies is, of course, that because believers have everlasting life in their new bodies they don't get sick either. Just as decay and death go together, equally health and everlasting life go together. It is inconceivable that we will be sick in heaven! Paul writes to the Romans in Romans 8:19-24 explaining precisely what I have been describing:

> *"The creation waits in eager expectation for the sons of God to be revealed. For the creation was subjected to frustration, not by its own choice, but by the will of the one who subjected it, in hope, that the creation itself will be liberated from its* ***bondage to decay*** *and brought into the glorious freedom of the children of God.*
>
> *We know that the whole creation has been groaning as in the pains of childbirth right up to the present time. Not only so, but we ourselves, who have the firstfruits of the Spirit, groan inwardly as we wait eagerly for our adoption as sons,* ***the redemption of our bodies.****"*

It is quite clear that we are not going to get our new sickness-free resurrection bodies right now. As Paul writes in verse 25: *"we wait for it patiently."*

Because all creation is in bondage to decay, you will grow old, acquire wrinkles, change shape, and become increasingly prone to sickness. The Bible never promises eternal youth. Indeed Proverbs 31:30 on the perfect wife tells us, *"Charm is deceptive, and beauty is fleeting."*

We need to lay this foundation from Genesis and understand the Fall. Christians are not divinely immune from sickness, as we shall see later. Nor should you feel any guilt in consulting a doctor if you're sick. You are no worse than the rest of the human race. Of course you should seek God first about your sickness and what treatment to take.

After a ministry trip in Nigeria a few years ago I developed flu symptoms. I soldiered on at work. Eventually I saw a doctor who took some blood, but nothing showed up. I carried on, eventually collapsing into bed with a fever. I could scarcely stand up. More blood was taken and analysed. I had falcifirum malaria, the most dangerous type, which can kill you in 48 hours. I was duly taken to hospital, arriving with a blood pressure of 60 over zero. Zero means there isn't any to measure! My wife insisted I had immediate treatment or there might not be a patient to treat at all. I was given the corrective treatment and duly recovered. I believe God spared my life and sustained me until I got proper medical treatment. I didn't blame the devil, or claim the automatic right to divine healing. I recognised that my human body is in bondage to decay, and needed corrective medical treatment. Certainly I was healed and even had to sign a government form to say I hadn't died!

Christians have been made to feel guilty for being sick and lacking in faith if they consult a doctor. Some have even denied they were sick at all and died as a result. The sensible Christian will strike the right balance between seeking God, prayer, common sense eating and exercise, and remembering that we are basically still under the curse of the Fall. Later we will cover what it means when Christ became a curse for us and redeemed us.

As we shall now see, the Fall is not the only source of sickness even though that was the gateway in. The effect was far reaching, affecting the animal kingdom also.

2

The Three Sources of Sickness

As we saw in the last chapter, the effects of the Fall of Man have continued for the last six thousand years, and the reality for everyone is that we all experience sickness to a greater or lesser degree. Even having a vaccination at birth proves the point. We are all vulnerable.

I am going to refer to sickness caused by the Fall and human frailty as physical sickness. For example, that was why Paul left Trophimas sick at Miletus (2 Timothy 4:20) and urged Timothy to take a little wine for his stomach's sake (1 Timothy 5:23). Basically he told him to stop drinking only water because the alcohol killed germs and water in hot countries is suspect. At this juncture I want to make a point which I am convinced is biblically correct and is also the key to knowing how to deal with sickness. There is a clear distinction between sicknesses which are **physical** in nature and origin and those which are **spiritual.** There is a third category where God Himself inflicts disease as a punishment on either individuals or a nation, and we will study those for the sake of completeness. If, like Herod, you take glory for yourself and are struck with worms (Acts 12:23) you won't get better by seeing the doctor. The cure will be good old-fashioned repentance before God!

The three sources of sickness can be simply stated as:

1) The Fall – physical

2) Satan – spiritual

3) God – judgement

We will now see how Satan, the devil, the father of lies, the accuser of the brethren, Apollyon, the destroyer, the dragon etc., fits into the picture.

As in Milton's Paradise Lost it's back to Genesis where it all started to go wrong. The physical decay was of course God's judgement on Adam and the whole human race, but Adam had more than a body. He had a spirit, which died the moment he sinned, and a soul. He therefore experienced three areas of change; sickness in his body, death in his human spirit, and bondage in his soul. But worst by far was that he was cut off from his fellowship with God. He was exposed, vulnerable and frightened. Suddenly he was now in the middle of a spiritual battle for the future of mankind itself. Satan (Lucifer) had been thrown down onto the earth (Isaiah 14:12) from his position in the heavens, with a third of the angels, and was out to destroy God's creation. The story can be read in Genesis 3, so I only want to draw attention to the consequences of the Fall where they affected Adam and Eve's souls.

First of all their eyes were opened. What does this mean? Clearly they could see physically, but suddenly they could see spiritually also. They were aware of the whole spiritual dimension, which hitherto God had kept from them. They had, as it were, been blind to it. Now they realised they were naked. Innocence was gone forever. Some areas of the spirit realm are out of bounds for everyone. These are most commonly called 'occult' (or hidden), and anyone who strays into these areas, intentionally or not, will be affected, possibly with physical sickness, as we shall see.

From awareness came guilt; from guilt came a covering over to conceal the nakedness; then the passing on of blame.

The attack against Man was on – against his soul, his mind, his will and his emotions. Invisible spirits (demons) would incite, exploit, and if they could, invade Man's soul. They were using their legal position to execute the curse God had pronounced on Man. Worse, it was possible for these curses to cross generation after generation down through the bloodline.

> *'He by no means clears the guilty, visiting the iniquity of the fathers on the children **to the third and fourth generation.**'*
> (Numbers 14:18 NKJV)

It is really important to understand this. We all have two parents, four grandparents, eight great-grandparents, and sixteen great-great-grandparents, making **thirty** people who affect us spiritually.

The likelihood that they were all godly and righteous saints is somewhat improbable, so there could be a curse which passes on down the family line. Examples would include a high incidence of cancer occurring in the family even though it is medically a non-hereditary disease. So, you cannot pass it on physically, but spirits of cancer may run in families which, for instance, practise Freemasonry, thus illustrating how it can be passed on spiritually. The incidences of a link between cancer and Freemasonry are far too frequent to ignore or put down as a statistical quirk. That's why Jesus healed the sick (physical) and cast out demons (spiritual), even if they manifested physically as with the woman with the bent back.

The text is very clear: she had had a spirit of infirmity for eighteen years, was bent over, and could in no way raise herself up (see Luke 13:11). Jesus told her *"Woman, you are loosed from your infirmity."* Note that He didn't say healed. It was a spiritual bondage manifesting physically, from which she was released. Jesus made it clear to the ruler of the synagogue when he argued, that Satan had bound her. We're not told why, but there was a moment in time eighteen years previously when access was gained by Satan to afflict her body.

I believe it is essential with God's help to recognise and discern the root cause of sickness correctly. There are countless cases of people being sick with no apparent medical cause. Doctors often refer to psychosomatic illnesses. That literally means 'disease of the soul' (psyche). It is recognised that well over half of all medical consultations fall into this category! They affect both **soul** and **body.**

The third source of sickness is when God Himself pronounces judgement. This is for those who reject His ways and is the outworking of His curse on mankind. This may sound odd. Indeed people ask how a God of love can do such things. The Deuteronomy 28 covenant with Israel sets out the choices: Obedience and blessing… or … disobedience and cursing. Some of the curses the Jews (God's special chosen people) could receive were plagues (verse 21), consumption/tuberculosis, inflammation and swelling, burning fever (malaria?) (verse 22), boils, tumours (cancer), with the scab and with the itch, from which you cannot be healed (verse 27), madness, blindness, confusion of heart (panic attacks) (verse 29). No use blaming the devil here, or indeed seeing the doctor! It required repentance from their wicked ways. That's still true. God hasn't changed, even if grace is extended because His compassion is over all that He has made (Psalm 145:8-9). Take AIDS, for example. God has immense compassion on men who are so wounded that they desperately seek male friendship and relationship. Yet those who practise an active homosexual lifestyle may receive in their bodies the due **penalty.** Romans 1:27 is clear:

> '...likewise the men ... burned with lust for one another, men with men committing what is shameful, and receiving in themselves the **penalty** of their error.'

I've heard testimonies of God healing AIDS patients, and I believe it can happen. He is the Almighty and we can draw down His mercy, but if people kept God's laws of monogamous marriage, this problem would disappear. That doesn't mean Christians don't care. Many selflessly devote their lives to teaching, care, and hospice work. The point I'm trying to make is that the answer is good old-fashioned biblical repentance for violating God's laws, not more medical research to protect people from the consequences Romans 1 describes. We break God's laws at our peril.

There are many examples in the Bible of God sending sickness as judgement. The plagues of Egypt would be a clear example. Interestingly barrenness is also attributed to God. 'The Lord closed the womb' we are told. See Genesis 20:18 (Sarah) and 1 Samuel 5 (Hannah).

We need to understand that God has laws of cause and effect, which operate not just in the natural realm but in the spiritual realm also. We know of many women pronounced medically incapable of conceiving and carrying to full term by the best specialists, yet who are now mothers. How? By identifying the root cause as a curse operating and breaking its power. Indeed I am the godparent of one such child, born after prayer to break the curse of barrenness. The point is simply this. The sickness/problem may be medical (physical). On the other hand it may not be, and if it does have a spiritual root, then by addressing the problem in prayer you may see a dramatic change. I would advise a full medical check first, but especially in cases where there is no apparent cause I would investigate further the possibility of a spiritual cause.

You can be spiritually 100% right with God and still be sick. Elisha had taken on Elijah's mantle, and received the double portion of the Spirit – something we'd all like. He saw Elijah taken up into heaven, yet 2 Kings 13:14 tells us:

> *'Now Elisha was suffering from the illness from which he died.'*

Even the prophet who God had used to heal others was himself equally vulnerable, and subject to the Fall. We need real discernment between the spiritual and the physical and to check both sources.

3

The Effects of the Curse

Unfortunately people identify a curse with swearing, when in reality it's the outworking of breaking God's laws, and facing the consequences.

The curse works at three levels:

a) On a nation
God's promise to Abraham remains valid (Genesis 12:3). He will curse those who curse Israel, and some nations are in the state they are in because of the way they have treated the Jews over the centuries. That's a whole area you can trace all through history, including Britain's since 1916.

b) On a family
As we've seen earlier, it can run down four generations. That's actually shorter than the curse of illegitimacy which runs for ten generations. In Deuteronomy 23:2 we're told someone with illegitimacy in his line was barred from entering the congregation. Nor were his children allowed in **for ten generations.** Why? Was it fair that children ten generations on paid the price for the sin of others? God says yes, because of the way that curse operates. It is generational in nature. If illegitimacy runs in a family there is a curse operating there, however much sociologists try to validate unbiblical common-law relationships. If there are any sicknesses which 'run in the family' it's living proof of the curse operating. You can read in the newspapers about curses in famous families.

c) On an individual
You may be affected by both the above if you live in a nation opposed to Israel, and come from a family where a hereditary (family) spirit has been wreaking havoc in everyone's lives. In Deuteronomy 27:14-28 the people were told what things would

bring a curse into their lives, and they had to say 'Amen' afterwards to show they understood and took it seriously. Galatians 3:10 reinforces this:

'For it is written: "Cursed is everyone who does not continue to do everything written in the Book of the Law".'

The good news for the Christian is that Jesus has freed us from the curse of the Law and we live under grace. For the unbeliever it is not so. They remain under the curse.

However freedom has to be appropriated like all of the benefits and blessings of salvation. If we remain in the words of Jesus we shall know the truth and the truth shall make us free from every curse operating in our lives. That's an individual's responsibility.

4

Christ our Redeemer

I hope we can now see the problem! We need to be freed from the effects of the Fall, the Curse, and its consequences. We understand that Jesus died for our sin, but it is essential to understand that He **also** became a curse for us. By becoming a curse Jesus paid the price for all the effects of the curse upon us and we need to appropriate that redemption by faith.

> *'Christ has redeemed us from the curse of the law, having become a curse for us (for it is written "Cursed is everyone who hangs on a tree").'* (Galatians 3:13)

We exchanged our sin and the effects of the sin (the curse) for His righteousness and the effects of it (forgiveness, restoration, health and wholeness).

That is the key Christians need to know.

This is the key to health and healing. We are redeemed (bought) from the curse.

Unfortunately the white Western education system of secular humanism denies the reality of such things even existing, but if you're reading this in Africa or Asia you will know immediately the reality of what I'm talking about and the power of curses. Alas, prosperous Western nations deny the reality of the spiritual realm and seek to rationalise everything in purely scientific terms. Jesus spoke of these things a great deal.

I now want to home in on the specifics of how to deal with sickness. This is addressed to the believer. For the unbeliever it's actually different. Indeed it's often easier for God to heal the unbeliever than the believer! Why? Because God will extend grace and mercy to show the unbeliever that he is loved, and that the gospel is true. In other words it's 'power evangelism'; preaching the gospel with signs following to prove it is true, and bringing sinners to repentance. That's why in Mark 16 the disciples and early believers were told to do just that: *'heal the sick... cast out demons.'* It's why people came to Jesus, and it should be why people come to us as well. That's why we hear of spectacular miracles at mass evangelistic rallies. I have seen it myself in India, with lepers healed, paralytics walking, the deaf hearing and the dumb speaking. And these people were Hindus! That's the power of healing and is, I believe, an important part of evangelism. The world is tired of philosophy and religion. They want to see something real and true, and God will confirm His word with signs **following** the preaching of the word. That's why I think every healing service needs to have the gospel preached first, so the signs (healing etc.) can follow! It brings faith and honours God.

However, for the believing Christian God paradoxically requires more. He requires repentance, changed behaviour and forgiveness of others. The rules are not the same as for the unbeliever. So we have unconditional power healing for the unbeliever to lead him to repentance, yet healing for the believer is often conditional.

For example, if I regard iniquity in my heart the Lord will not hear me (Psalm 66:18), and indeed 1 Peter 3:7 makes it clear that if you're in contention with your wife your prayers will be hindered.

Too often believers expect God to just ignore their sin, their attitudes and their behaviour, and heal them even when they violate the most basic principles of repentance, faith, forgiveness of others etc.

Wrong thinking like this leads to disappointment and discredits the gospel. A basic starting point when we go to meetings should be to be totally right with God and one another. God requires us to walk in the light – no skeletons in the cupboard, and to walk in truth – no deception of others, or indeed ourselves. Openness is required. *'Confess your sins to one another and pray for one another that you may be healed'* (James 5:16).

If every healing meeting had a confession time first, I'm sure we'd see more folk healed. We cannot ignore the Scriptures and simply hope God will be nice to us if He's in a good mood, or it's a good day for the preacher. Even if you get healed through faith operating, it'll be very hard to retain it.

How many people suffer from arthritis because they will not forgive?

How many people are sick due to bad relationships?

Relationships have to be put right. Indeed, Jesus says they have to be put right **before** going to church, and **before** coming into the presence of God.

> *'Therefore, if you are offering your gift at the altar and there remember that your brother has something against you, leave your gift there in front of the altar. First go and be reconciled to your brother; then come and offer your gift.'*
>
> (Matthew 5:23-24)

It is that important. You cannot offer up an acceptable sacrifice of praise, while others have things against you that you know about and need to be put right. Only then will you really have the boldness and assurance of faith to ask what you want of God with a clean heart (Hebrews 10:19-22).

In most churches there are usually a number of unresolved relationship difficulties, which could block healing.

God wants to deal with the cause, not just the effect. It's your soul He wants to heal, as well as your body. So we need to see what's physical and what's spiritual, and the root cause.

5

Physical or Spiritual?

To begin with we need to affirm the totality of our salvation, that Jesus died for every sin of every person, and His sacrifice fully paid the price. We are truly redeemed from every sin, every sickness, every curse, and we need to understand the glory, the fullness and the totality of what God in Christ did for us. It is truly awesome; not just dealing with the sin problem but far, far more. ==We are ransomed, healed, restored and forgiven.== Amazing grace indeed! If Jesus had not redeemed us from the Curse, or indeed died for our sickness, which is a result of the Fall, our salvation would be incomplete. The name Jesus in Hebrew actually means **God heals** as well as **God saves.** His very name proclaims His victory over sickness. If you believe in Jesus you believe in **'God heals'.** That's His name. It's truly marvellous.

In His role as the second Adam He restored all that was lost, even if we do not yet see all the benefits of that restoration here and now on earth.

Hebrews 2:8 tells us:

> *'For in that He put all in subjection under Him (Jesus), He left nothing that is not put under him. But we do not **yet** see all things put under him. But we see Jesus.'*

In other words, although everything is under the Lord's feet it's not all yet fully revealed. We have to wait (Romans 8:22-25).

Some physical sicknesses will be obvious, including accidents, broken bones, birth deformities, colds, flu etc. A very good rule of thumb is this: if it's a medically recognised treatable condition it most likely has a straight physical cause. God has physical laws for the human body for our welfare and protection. The human body is designed to heal itself. It has antibodies; and we are indeed fearfully and wonderfully made (Psalm 139:14).

If you are permanently disabled through an accident your body may be unable to heal itself. You may need a special creative miracle by God. I recently heard of a recreated knee joint, which totally baffled the specialists as the old X-rays showed irreparable damage but the new one showed a perfect knee.

God's will is that we are well, and He uses His physical laws to achieve that. Most medical sicknesses now are curable with a few exceptions, which include viruses, and the common cold. Sick Christians sometimes give up too quickly, assuming it must be God's will that they're sick. That flows from wrong reasoning, which says that God is sovereign, therefore God's will is always done. I'm sick, so that must be God's will. Wrong! The flaw in the argument is that God's will is always done. That is just not so. God's will is that everyone is saved and that none should perish as 2 Peter 3:9 clearly tells us. But clearly many will. So God's will is **not** done, in that sense. Yes, He remains sovereign, but works within spiritual laws. That's also true of healing.

Some who assert it's God's will for them to be sick actively seek to get out of God's will – if they really believed it to be so – by seeing their doctor. Of course God wants us to get well. We need to move beyond passive simplistic acceptance of sickness as something we just have to accept and live with.

Spiritual or spirit-based sickness is harder to pinpoint. For example headaches can be either, as can migraine, backache, stomach pain and what in India they call 'body weakness': they just feel ill all over!

However a number of spirit-based diseases are mentioned in the Bible:

A spirit of infirmity (Luke 13:11)
This is a demonic attack of a non-specific sickness. If something is around you get it. Doctors can't identify any cause. You're sickness-prone and it's one thing after another. Alas it's all too common. The most common manifestations are backache and oppressive headaches. There has to be a gateway in for it to operate.

A spirit of heaviness (Isaiah 61:3)
Also called depression. It can be medically caused, as in post-natal depression, and it's estimated that 20% of the population may have a chemical imbalance affecting behaviour, but here we're talking about a spirit bringing that heavy weight of oppression, darkness, suicidal thoughts etc. Jesus quotes this passage in Luke 4. If you discern the cause is demonic, encourage the sufferer to fill their house with the sounds of praise. Their spirit will be fed and the oppression should lift, just as it did when David played for King Saul.

Familiar spirits (Leviticus 19:31)
These run through families and have knowledge of past family members. They operate with psychic powers. Some people mistakenly believe these powers are from God. Others go to spiritualist 'churches' where familiar spirits operate.

Other spirits mentioned are an unclean spirit (Mark 1:23), a dumb spirit (Mark 9:17), a spirit of divination (Acts 16:16), as well as more general references to evil spirits.

So how do you tell? You need the gift of discernment, and to ask God for a word of knowledge or a word of wisdom as to why someone is ill. An evangelist told me about a lady who was constantly sick. He prayed and asked God why the lady remained sick and was told 'It's the water'. The lady got a water filter and couldn't believe what it filtered out. It was like frogspawn. After that she recovered quite quickly. It was a straight problem of poisons and toxins in her water, revealed by a word of knowledge. God really does know the answer.

In her case they started thinking it was a spiritual attack, but God showed it was physical, and the opposite can also be true. We mustn't jump to conclusions. We need wisdom from above to discern correctly, based on the presenting problem.

6

Biblical Methods of Healing

Although Jesus used many different methods of healing, from just speaking the word to making paste for a man's eyes, I believe there are three main methods given to the Church.

a) *The Laying on of hands*
This is based on Mark 16, and is, I believe, for unbelievers as well, repeating the ministry of Jesus.

The promise is that they shall recover. This is important as it implies a process of time. An instant healing is more accurately the working of a miracle. It's important to differentiate to avoid an unbiblical expectation.

The first time I received prayer for a longstanding condition I felt nothing specific change. Nor was I better the next day. But over a 6 week period the condition cleared up and hasn't recurred for 25 years. That's biblical healing – over time. Sometimes I meet someone who asks me if I remember praying for them 6 months ago. They then tell me they are healed now. These were not conditions which would have got better, they were major longstanding illnesses! Wait for God to complete the work, and for full recovery.

b) *Summoning the Elders*
I believe the pattern in the Church should be:
i) Consult your doctor. There is nothing unspiritual in this. Take whatever medicine is prescribed.
ii) At the same time pray for yourself. Ask God to show you why you are sick and how He intends to heal you.
iii) If you're still not better after i) and ii) get others to pray for you, such as those in your house group.
iv) If you're still not getting better apply James 5:14 and get your elders to anoint you with oil.

They are not an emergency service to rush round immediately, but are there to pray for you as God's order and remedy.

Note again, it's the prayer of faith, linked to forgiveness of sins. You should have confessed all sins to God and thoroughly repented before you send for the elders. Verse 16 is as important as verse 15.

c) *Gifts of healing/special meetings*
God has given gifts into the Body of Christ, but believers must go to those meetings properly prepared to receive. These meetings are the preferred route of many, judging by attendance. We want God's man of faith and power and anointing to do it all. It's what I call the Naaman expectation. He was angry when told to do something. It wasn't what he'd come for.

> *'Indeed I said to myself, "He will surely come out to me, and stand and call on the name of the Lord his God, and wave his hand over the place, and heal the leprosy".'*
> (2 Kings 6:11)

Is that your expectation? Has God told you to do something? I know of a businessman who wouldn't pay a debt he owed. When he got into the healing line God gave the evangelist a word of knowledge. His refusal to pay was blocking his healing. It was sin. He went away, paid the debt and was healed. There's a lesson there.

I'm personally keen on special meetings, but they must be done biblically. There must be teaching on repentance, confession, forgiving one another and being in right relationships. That paves the way for gifts of healing to flow unhindered, with words of knowledge, plus faith.

We must go properly prepared to really benefit from such meetings, being right with God and right with each other.

7

Blockages to Healing

It's clear we're part of the fallen human race, and we're decaying day by day. But God has redeemed us and given us the firstfruits of a glorious inheritance.

It's not a question of just claiming the promises or rebuking the devourer, but rather discerning what's happening and pulling down those strongholds and every power that would oppose God.

There can be real strongholds to overcome. The most common are:

Unforgiveness and resentment
Many sick people have been really hurt emotionally. They are wounded and all churned up inside. This will manifest in all sorts of ways from stress to rashes to blood conditions to arthritis. I believe such people need God's help to forgive. Yes, the Bible tells us we must forgive others to receive God's forgiveness, and unforgiveness is a blockage. It may take time. If you identify with this I would suggest first focusing prayer on the hurt, then on the sickness. Don't let it take root (Hebrews 12:15).

Occult strongholds
If you have violated major spiritual laws and entered forbidden satanic territory there can be a terrible price to pay. But once you're saved you have the right to be totally free from the effects of these areas, if you have repented and renounced them. This needs to be done before healing prayer. We must verbally renounce all occultic ties, laying the axe to the root. That includes horoscopes, ouija boards, fortune telling, tarot cards and even some artifacts in the home which may be picked up innocently. Anything ungodly must be removed. From experience I would include prayer for tattoos, and New Age and occultic jewellery, however fashionable.

Hereditary Curses
We have covered familiar spirits operating in a family, through the bloodline. Does anything run in your family? Cancer? Freemasonry? Heart attacks? Divorce? Miscarriages? Barrenness? In my case it was Christian Science and heart attacks. We need to repent and renounce all involvement, wilful or not.

Unbelief/wrong teaching
If Jesus could do nothing in Nazareth because of unbelief we're unlikely to do any better, and there's a lot about! Wrong teaching and exaggerated claims have created false expectations. Solid biblical teaching will release faith.

> *'Paul, observing him intently and **seeing he had faith to be healed,** said with a loud voice "Stand up straight on your feet"!'* (Acts 14:9)

Sometimes in the healing line it's right to ask someone 'Do you have faith?' If the answer is not really, then pray for the gift of faith (1 Corinthians 12:9). I've seen that produce healing more effectively than praying irrespectively. God will not work in unbelief. Whatever is not of faith is sin (Romans 14:23) and God will not work other than in the faith realm.

God does not want to block our healing. So if it's not appearing it's quite reasonable to ask why! Words of knowledge and gifts of discernment are there for the Church to be able to overcome these obstacles and see the results we all want.

8

What to do if You're Sick

- Identify what sickness you have and its likely cause. That may mean consulting your doctor to get a proper diagnosis.

- Get proper treatment and co-operate by taking any medication you are prescribed.

- At the same time pray and ask God to show you if your sickness is caused by any other factor than the basic fall of mankind, and a recognition that we are all in bondage to decay and the ageing process.

For example, are you discerning the body and blood of the Lord Jesus Christ correctly? (1 Corinthians 11:29). Paul tells the believers that because they are doing it in an unworthy manner, i.e. without having repented properly, they are bringing judgement on themselves in the form of sickness. As **many** were sick and some had died, it was clearly a common problem. If it was common then, we cannot discount it now.

Not discerning the body simply means that you are abusing the fact that Jesus died for you by continuing in wilful sin, and if you continue the result may well be sickness, even sickness unto death (1 Corinthians 11:30).

Persistent refusal to acknowledge sin of any kind and turn away from it may well lead to sickness in varying forms.

It does not necessarily follow that if you're sick that's the reason, but a Christian out of fellowship forfeits God's protection, and I have seen this. I have also seen it in cases where people refuse to heed a prophetic warning from God.

I believe the key is a right relationship with God and with one another. Because we all fall short of God's standard we need to identify areas of spiritual vulnerability and confess and renounce any possible occultic activity and other gateways into our lives including such common practises as fortune-telling and reading horoscopes in the daily newspaper.

However, we're all vulnerable, so what if you're diagnosed with a major illness, potentially terminal? In addition to the above I would suggest a time of prayer and fasting.

There are three things which always touch God's heart; repentance, humility, and fasting. He has a heart of compassion, grace, love and mercy. I firmly believe in the promises of God, but don't like the approach of commanding God to heal me.

I prefer to ask God for His mercy, grace and healing, not as a 'right', but as a blessing of sonship.

Repentance
This is so fundamental to healing, yet is not included in many meetings. 1 John 1:9 is the key:

> *'If we confess our sins, He is faithful and just to forgive us our sins and to cleanse us from all unrighteousness.'*

It has two parts – forgiveness **and** cleansing.

God is absolutely faithful to forgive us when we confess our sin. He knows us through and through, but still requires this of us. It **will** affect how He views us.

Humility
God always notes those who humble themselves. For example, when Ahab was told of judgement he humbled himself.

God actually said to Elijah *'Do you see how Ahab has humbled himself before me? Because he has humbled himself before me I will not bring the calamity in his days'* (1 Kings 21:29). God resists the proud but gives grace to the humble.

'Therefore humble yourselves under the mighty hand of God' (1 Peter 5:5-6). Humility gets God's attention.

Fasting
In Isaiah 58:6-8 God describes the fast He's looking for. Please

read it if you're sick! The conclusion is:

> *'Then shall your light break forth like the morning, **your healing shall spring forth speedily.**'* (Isaiah 59:8)

There is a fast for healing. We can influence God!

Jesus said we should never give up. Keep praying, keep asking, keep knocking.

Jesus is the same yesterday, today, and forever (Hebrews 13:8) and divine healing definitely didn't cease with the early Church. Indeed testimonies run all through Church history.

Should everyone be healed? I believe that is possible if we had all the knowledge, all the keys, and all the faith. Sometimes God's answer is no, as with Paul's thorn in the flesh, but he got his answer from God. We need to know the mind of the Lord, but until God specifically says no (and Paul was given the reason), then I believe we should continue to pray and expect to get better. We should appeal to God for His mercy.

The principles outlined above are well illustrated in 2 Kings chapter twenty. Hezekiah was sick. Actually he was going to die.

> Isaiah told him *"Thus saith the Lord; 'Set you house in order, for **you shall die,** and not live'."* (Verse 1)

That was a definite word from God.
But Hezekiah turned his face to the wall and prayed:

> *"'Remember now, O Lord, I pray, how I have walked before you in your sight.' And Hezekiah wept bitterly."*

That touched God's heart. God changed his mind! Isaiah hadn't even left the premises before God told him:

> *"Return and tell Hezekiah... I have heard your prayer, I have seen your tears; surely **I will heal you.**"*

God added 15 years to his life. Hezekiah had touched God's

heart. Note he went the medical route for his boil with a poultice of figs. No 'instant' healing there, but it is well worth studying the route Hezekiah took to obtain his healing. A good model is:

1. Confess all known sin.

2. Repent and renounce anything which you think might have caused the sickness.

3. Remind God of your service to Him.

4. Appeal to God's mercy, love and grace.

David writes in Psalm 103:

'Bless the Lord, O my soul,
And forget not all his benefits:
Who forgives all your iniquities,
*Who **heals all your diseases.**'*

He knew what we need to know. Right relationship with God and one another opens the way for God to work powerfully in our lives bringing maximum blessing and health.

Finally remember that the name **Jesus** means **God heals.** It's His name and it's His nature. He wants to do it for you.

'Call on Me in the day of trouble:
I will deliver you, and you shall glorify Me.'

(Psalm 50:15)

That's for this life. But for eternity God has promised us a new resurrection body. Paul describes this in 1 Corinthians 15. No more sickness, no more pain. Truly we shall be like Jesus, healed in spirit, soul, and body.

Finally... never give up

Sometimes it all seems so unfair. We've tried our best to serve God, yet still we're sick. We are basically people of faith, who trust in the Lord, yet may have an ongoing debilitating condition. What should we do? God is good, yet it can seem to us that He is not giving us the answer we need.

In Luke 18, Jesus told His disciples a parable to show them that they should **always pray and never give up.** He said:

> *"In a certain town there was a judge who neither feared God nor cared about men, And there was a widow in that town who kept coming to him with the plea, 'Grant me justice against my adversary.'*
>
> *"For some time he refused. But finally he said to himself, 'Even though I don't fear God or care about men, yet because this widow keeps bothering me I will see that she gets justice, so that she won't eventually wear me out with her coming!'*
>
> *"And the Lord said, 'Listen to what the unjust judge says. And will not God bring about justice for his chosen ones, who cry out to him day and night? Will he keep putting them off? I tell you, he will see that they get justice and quickly'."*

We need to invest our faith in praying positively and persistently to our Father in heaven, and never give up.

2 Peter 3:7 reminds us:

> *"The Lord is not slow in keeping his promise, as some understand slowness."*

It may take time, but we need to keep praying, particularly in the context of a church, where believers can bear one another's burdens. Jesus presences Himself in the midst, and we can apply the Word of God:

> *"Is any one of you in trouble? He should pray. Is anyone happy? Let him sing songs of praise. Is any one of you sick? He should call the elders of the church to pray over him and anoint him with oil in the name of the Lord.* ***And the prayer offered in faith will make the sick person well; the Lord will raise him up.*** *If he has sinned he will be forgiven.*
>
> *Therefore confess your sins to each other and **pray for each other so that you may be healed.**"*
>
> (James 5:15)

May the Word of God and faith bring you the healing you need, in the name of Jesus, whose very name means **'God heals'**.

Amen

If you have enjoyed this book and would like to help us to send a copy of it and many other titles to needy pastors in the **Third World**, please write for further information or send your gift to:

Sovereign World Trust, P.O. Box 777, Tonbridge, Kent TN11 0ZS, United Kingdom

or to the **'Sovereign World'** distributor in your country. If sending money from outside the United Kingdom, please send an International Money Order or Foreign Bank Draft in STERLING, drawn on a **UK** bank to **Sovereign World Trust**.